Yoga

Educise
EDUCATION & EXERCISE FOR KIDS
4 Kids

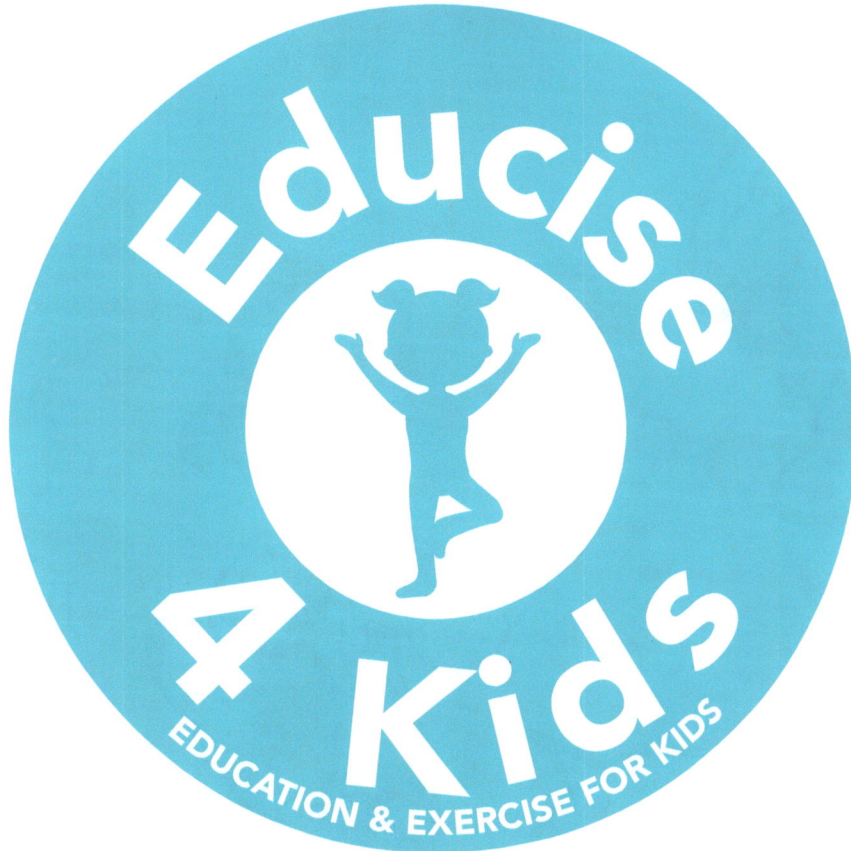

Created By
Priscilla Fauvette

Illustrated By
Bernard Fauvette

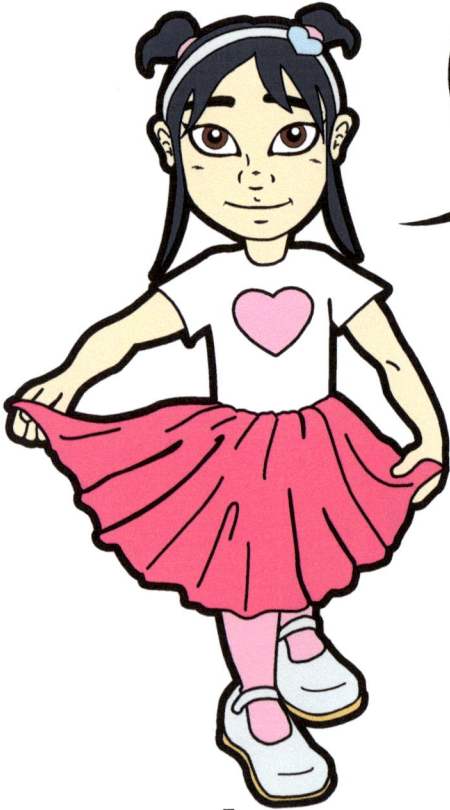

MAKE TIME FOR REST & RELAXATION

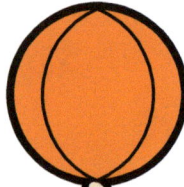

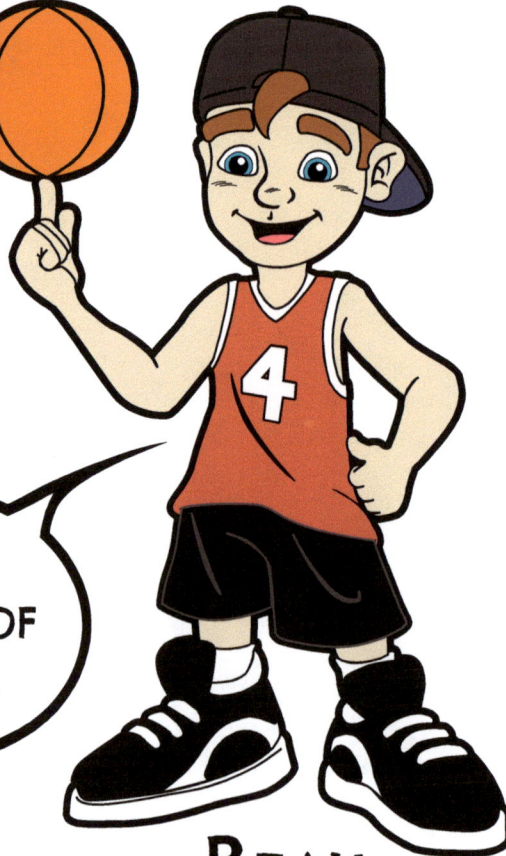

DRINK PLENTY OF WATER

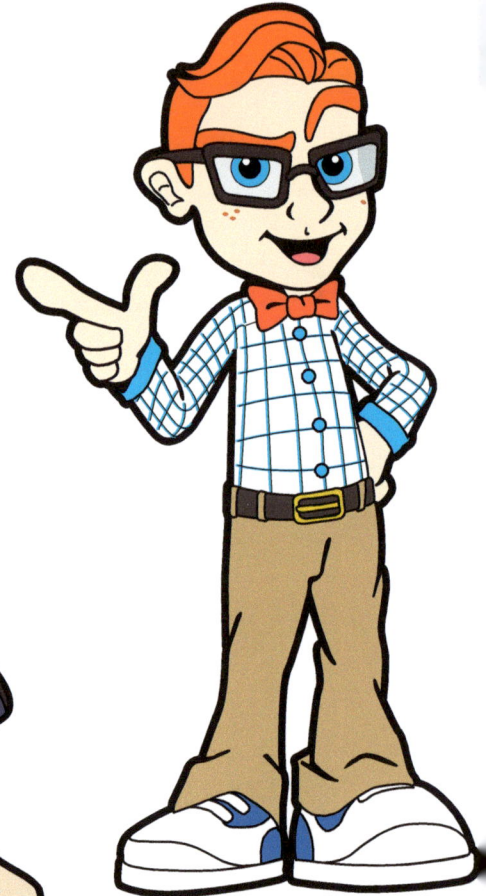

LIN

BEAU

CADEN

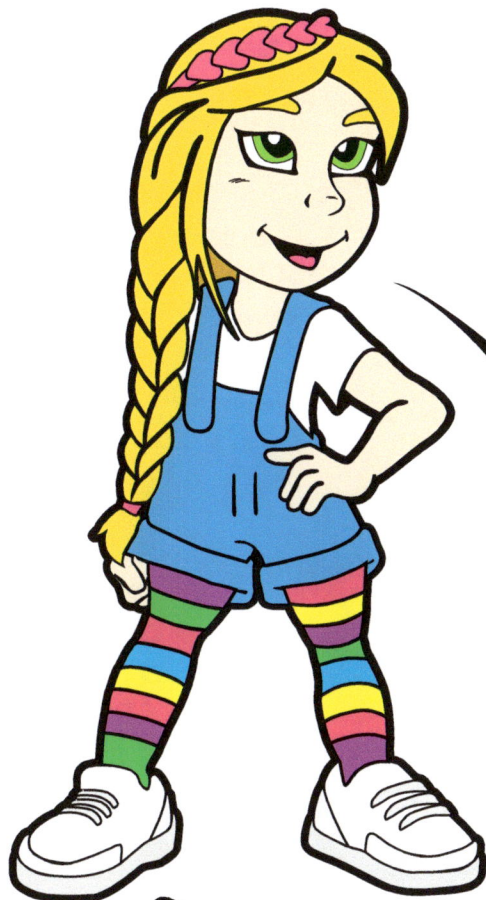

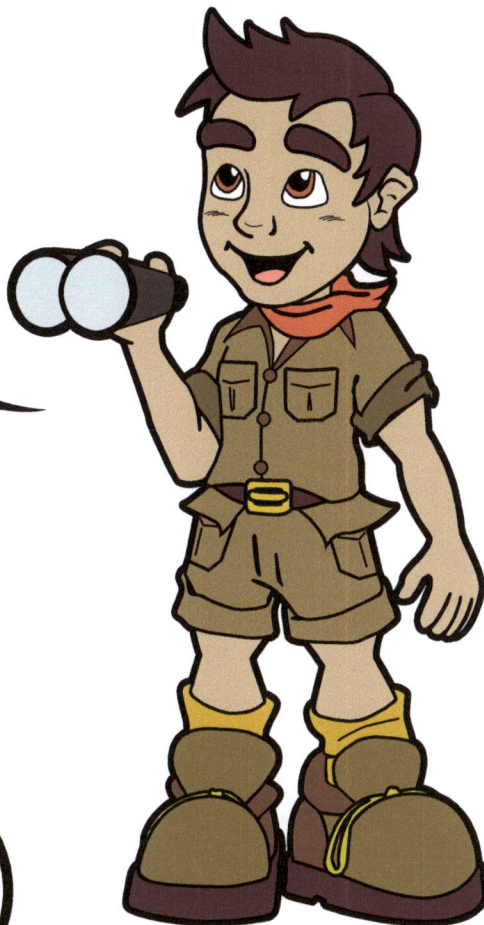

SOPHIE

ZAC

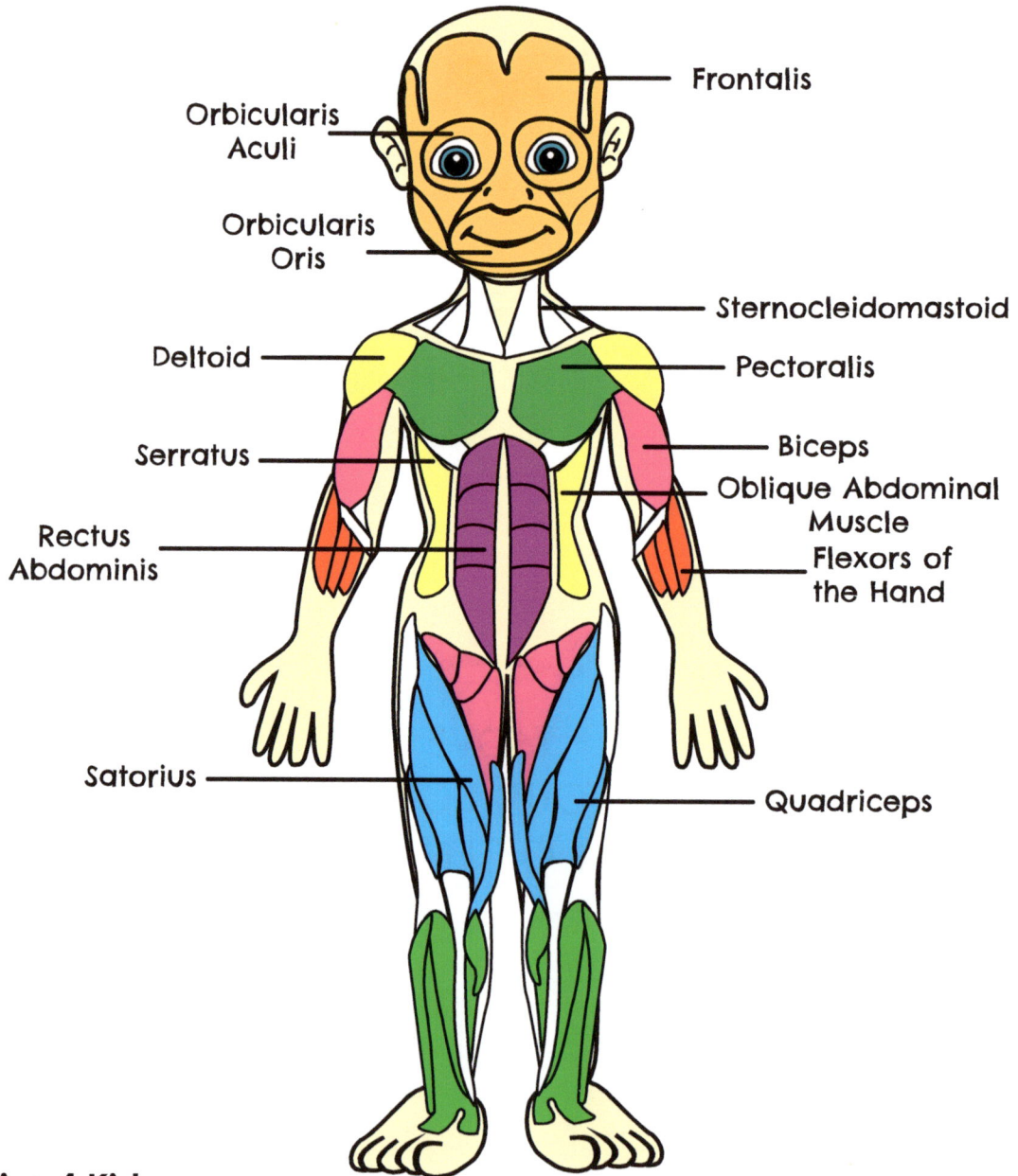

Anatomy

Frontalis

Orbicularis Aculi

Orbicularis Oris

Sternocleidomastoid

Deltoid

Pectoralis

Serratus

Biceps

Oblique Abdominal Muscle

Rectus Abdominis

Flexors of the Hand

Satorius

Quadriceps

Anatomy

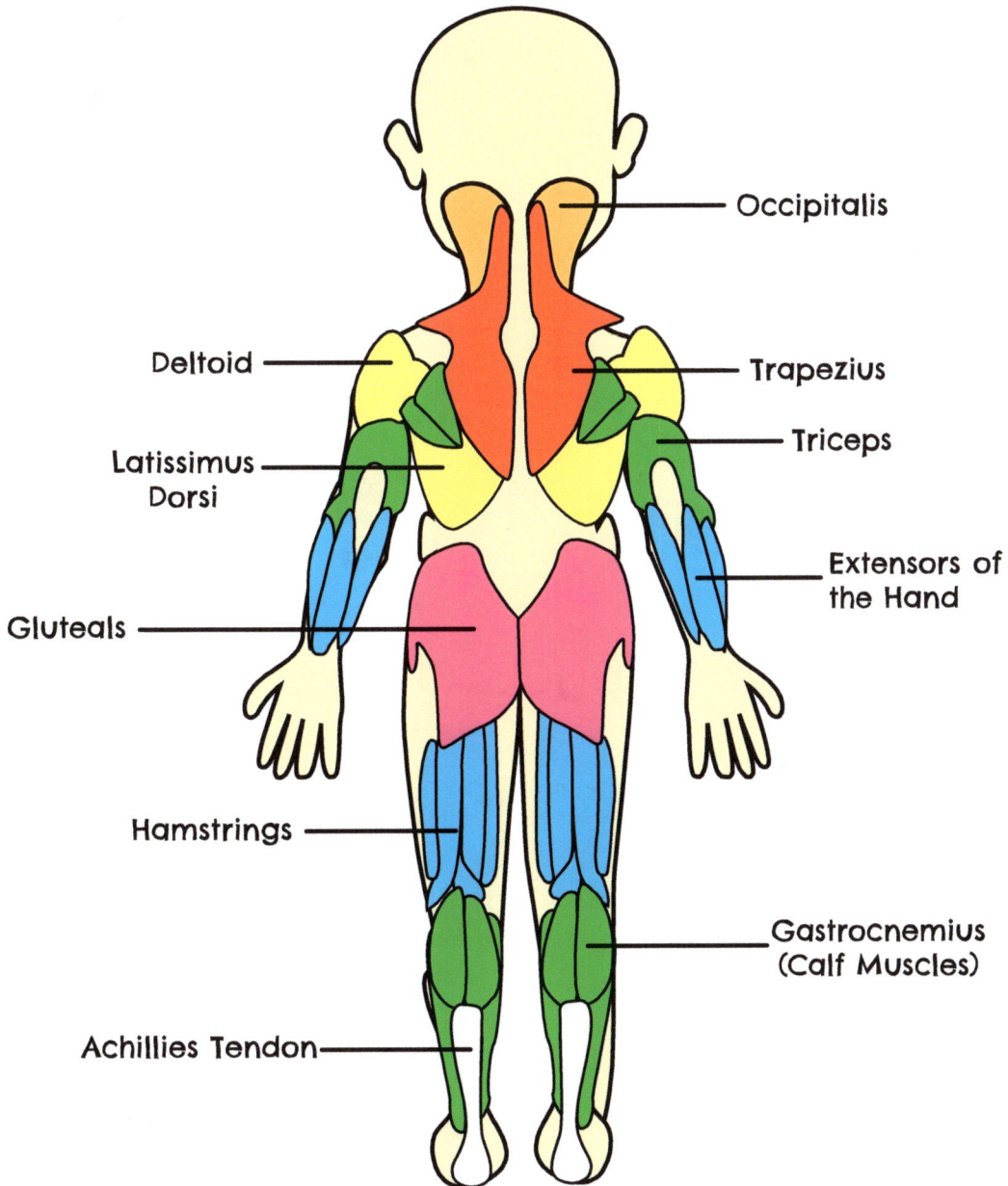

Occipitalis

Deltoid

Trapezius

Triceps

Latissimus Dorsi

Extensors of the Hand

Gluteals

Hamstrings

Gastrocnemius (Calf Muscles)

Achillies Tendon

Easy Pose

Sit on the floor

Cross your legs

Relax your back

Place your hands on your knees

Slowly breathe in and out

Hold this pose for 5 seconds

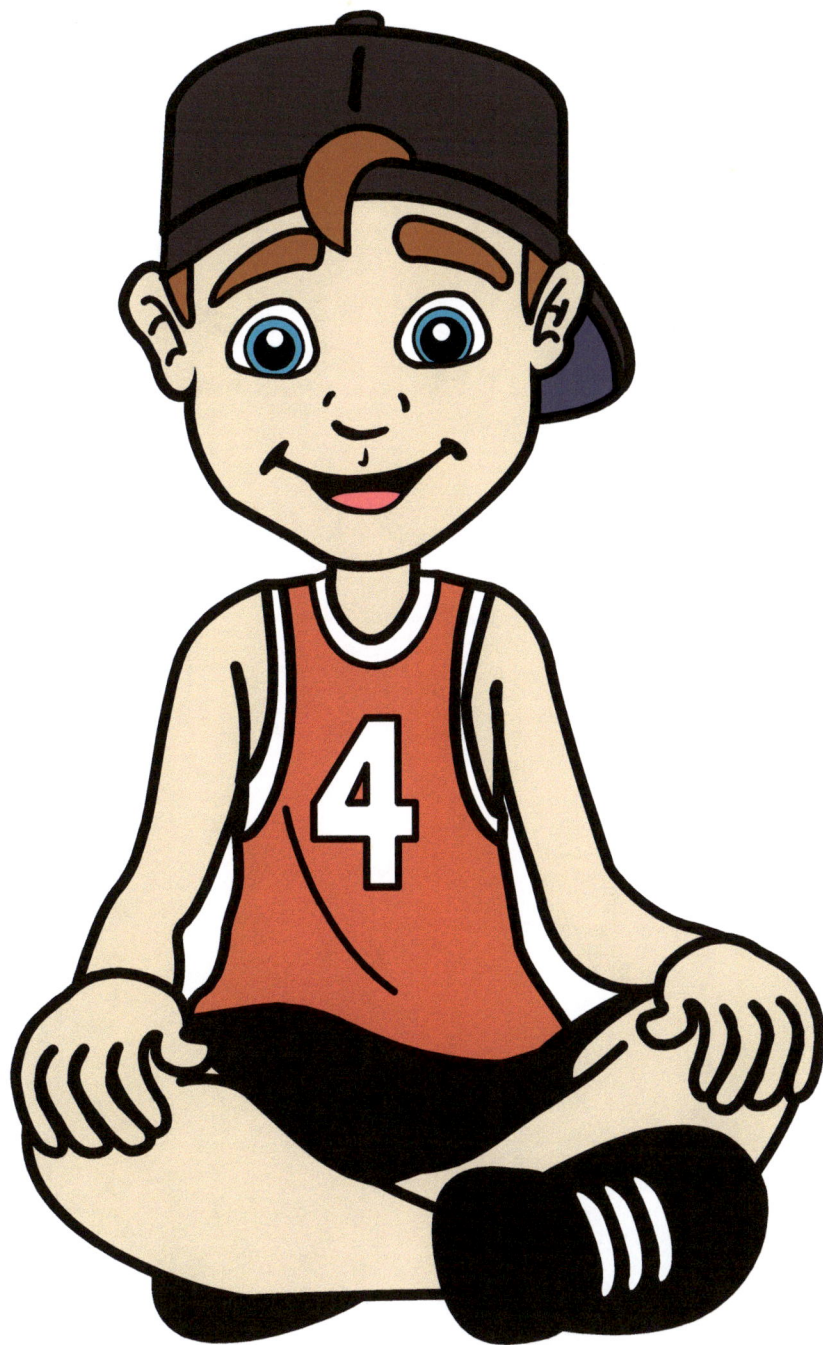

Cow Pose

Kneel on the floor
Put your palms on the floor
Slowly curve your back down
Slowly breathe in and out
Hold this pose for 5 seconds

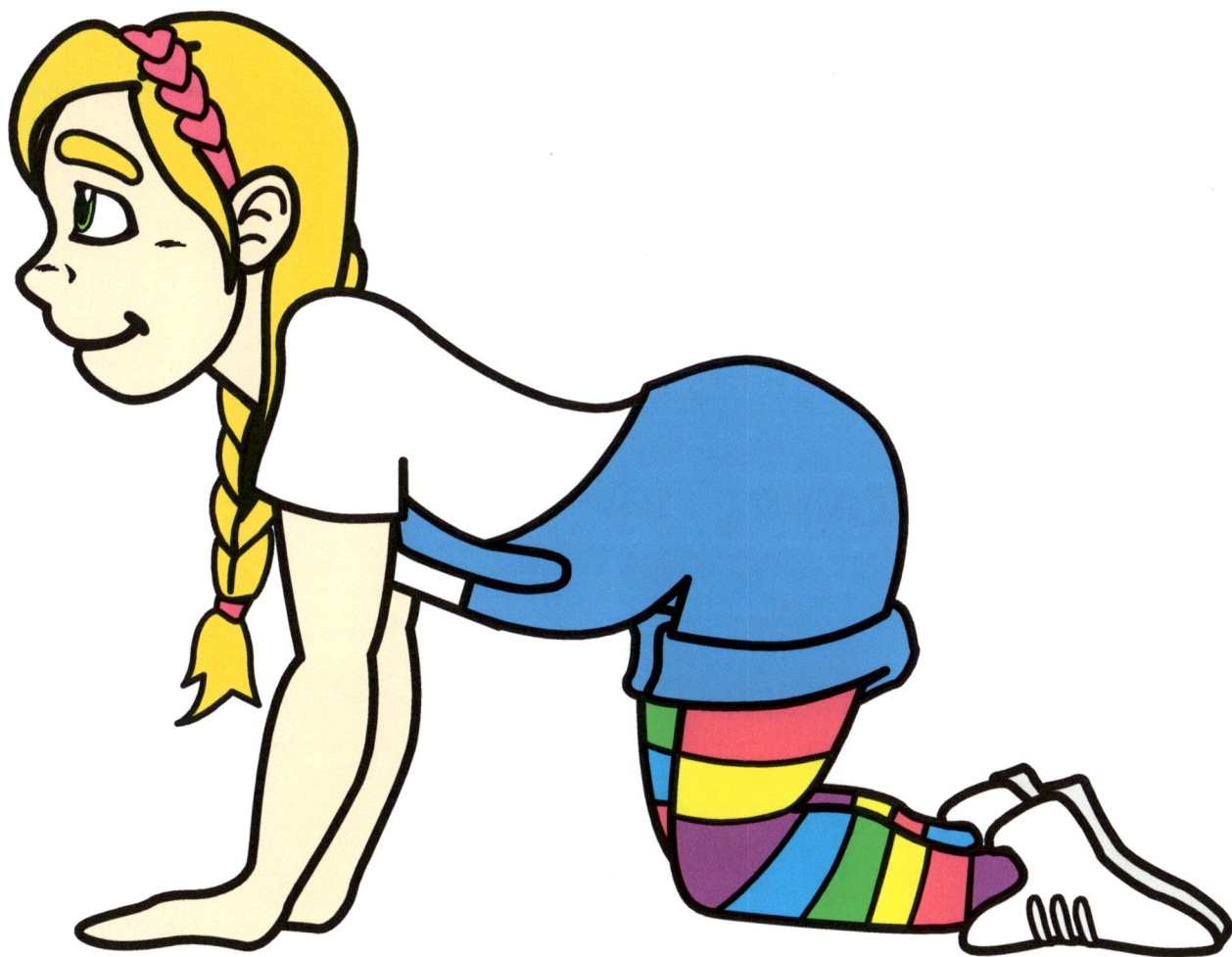

Half Moon Pose

Stand up straight

Point one toe to the side

Slowly lower one arm to the floor

Reach your other arm and leg up high

Slowly breathe in and out

Hold this pose for 5 seconds

Let's do this to the other side

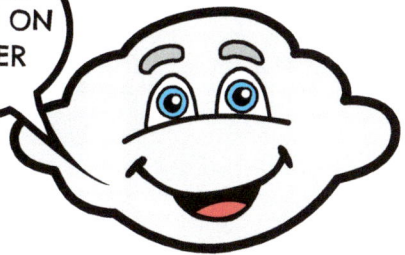

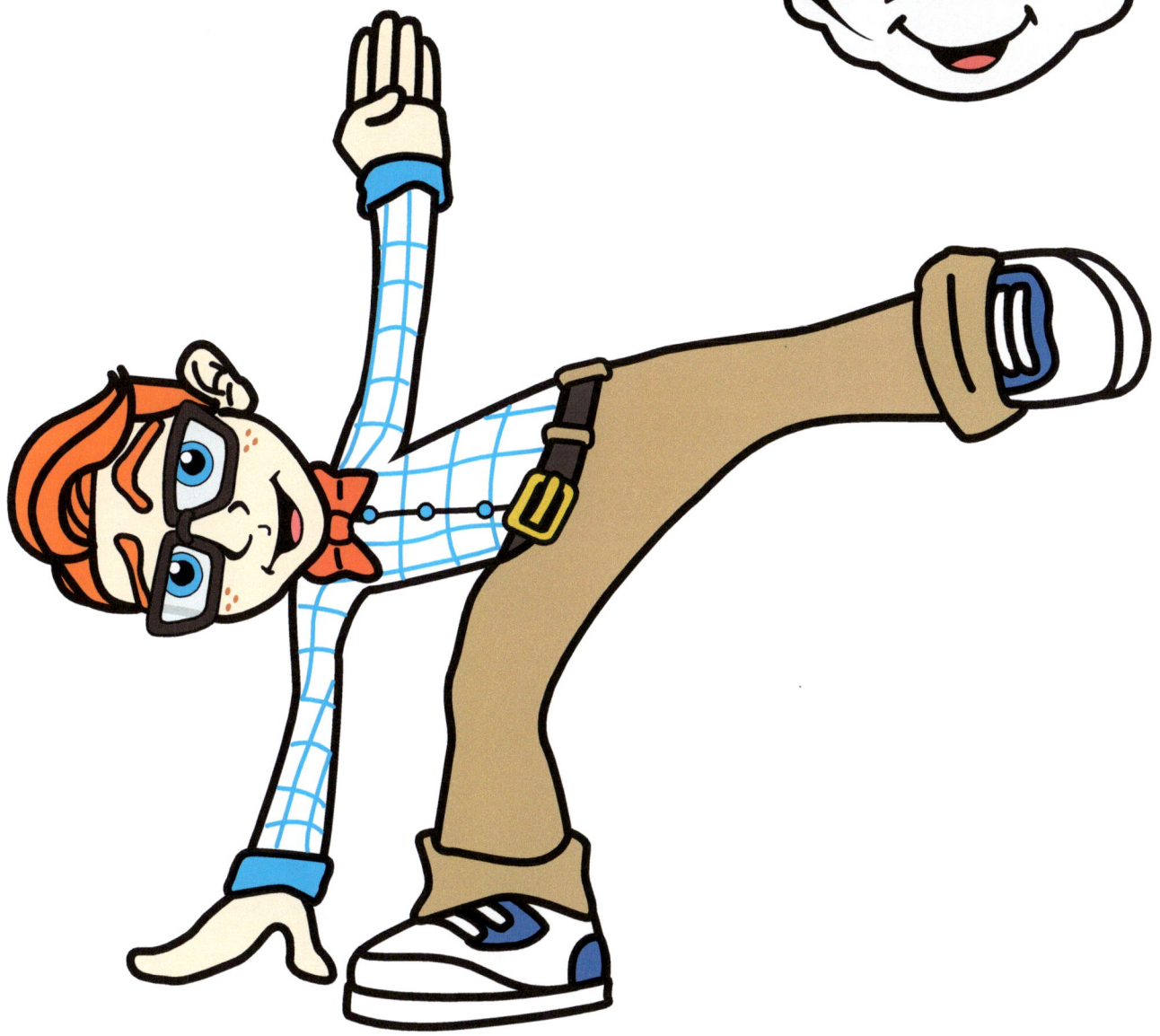

Tree Pose

Stand up straight

Slide one leg up

Place your left foot beside your knee

Lift your arms

Touch your palms together

Slowly breathe in and out

Hold this pose for 5 seconds

Let's do this to the other side

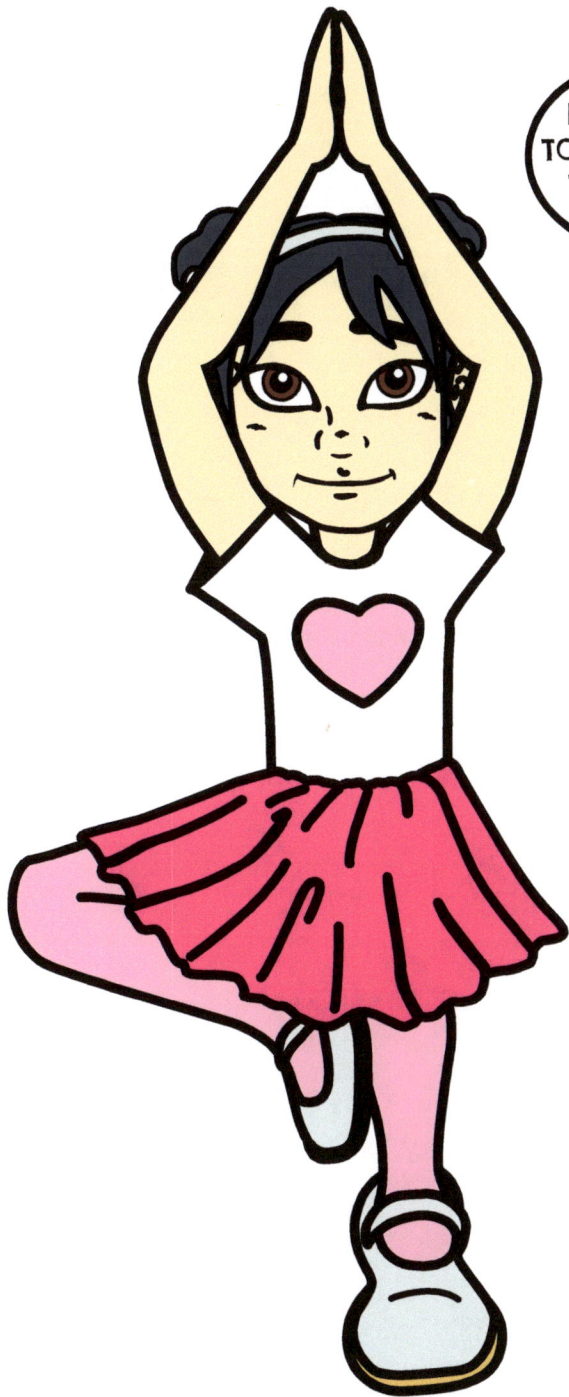
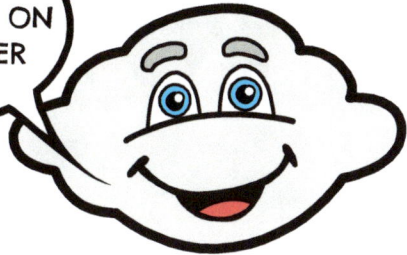

REMEMBER TO REPEAT ON THE OTHER SIDE

Warrior Pose

Stand up straight

Twist your body to the left

Take a step to the left

Point your toe

Lower your body

Slowly breathe in and out

Hold this pose for 5 seconds

Let's do this to the other side

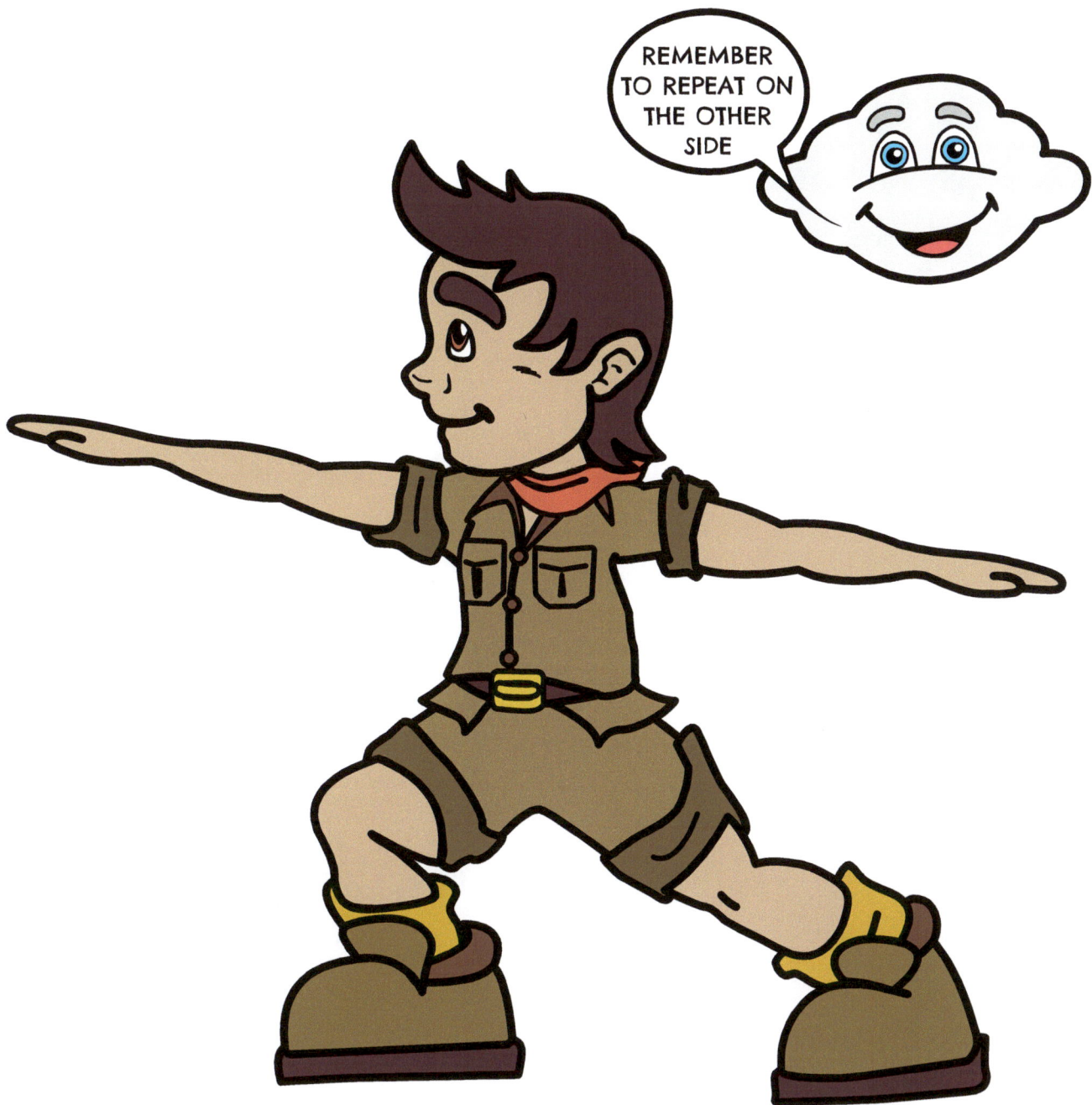

Plank Pose

Lay your stomach on the floor

Get up on your hands and toes

Keep your back straight

Slowly breathe in and out

Hold this pose for 5 seconds

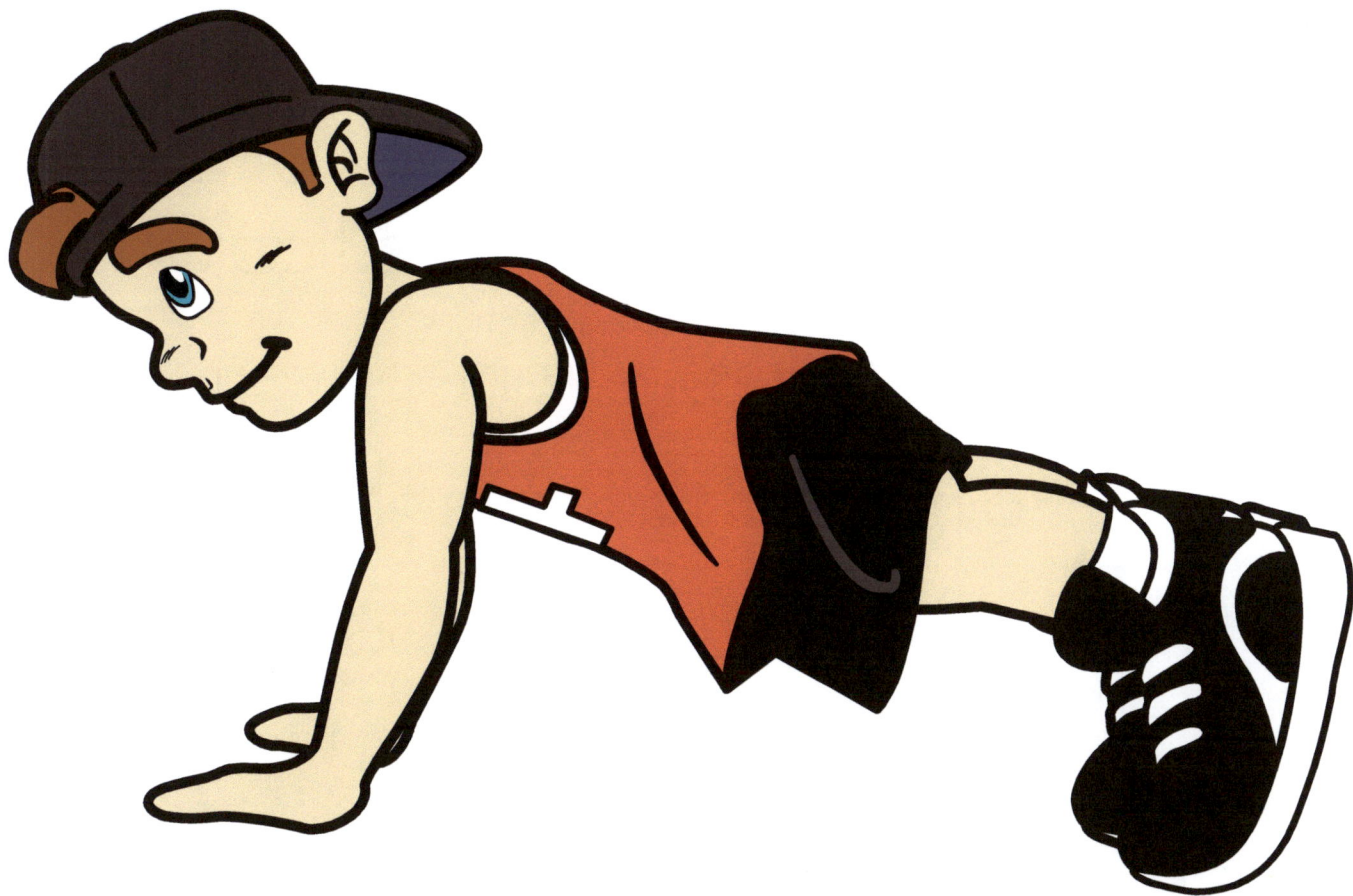

Upward Facing Dog Pose

Lay your stomach on the floor

Put your palms in front of you

Point your toes straight

Slowly push your upper body up

Curve your back

Slowly breathe in and out

Hold this pose for 5 seconds

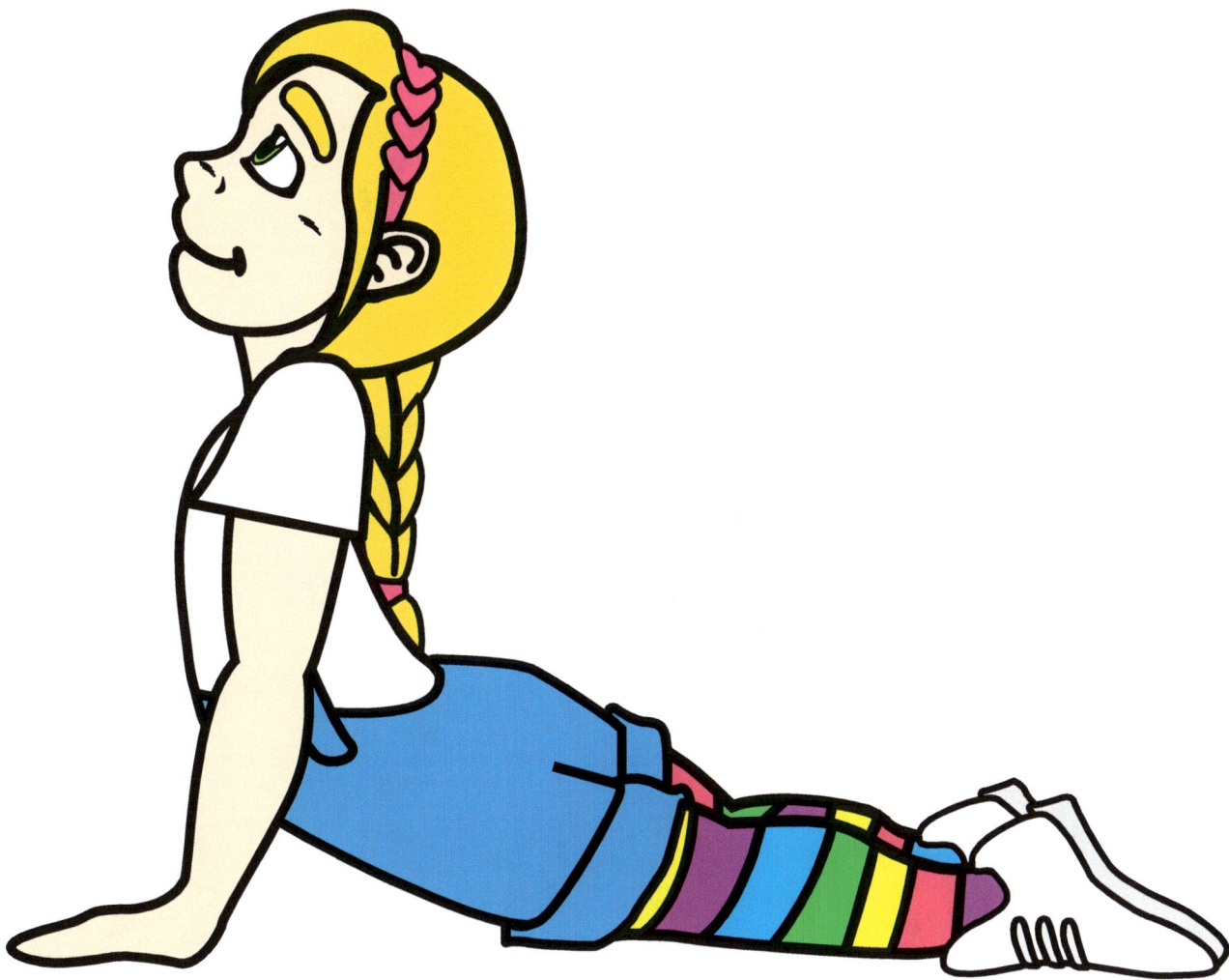

Cats Pose

Kneel on the floor
Put your palms on the floor
Slowly arch your back up
Slowly breathe in and out
Hold this pose for 5 seconds

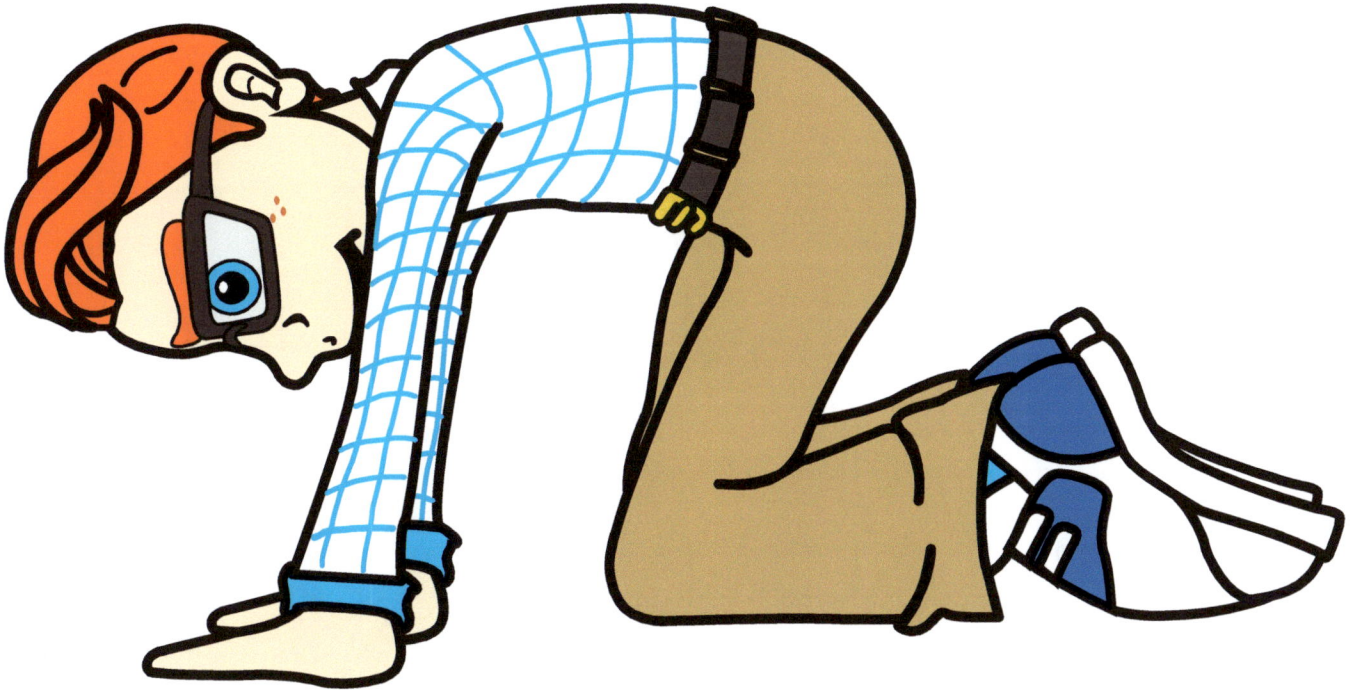

Yoga 21

Butterfly Pose

Sit on the floor

Place your feet together

Place your hands over your feet

Press your elbows onto your knees

Slowly breathe in and out

Hold this pose for 5 seconds

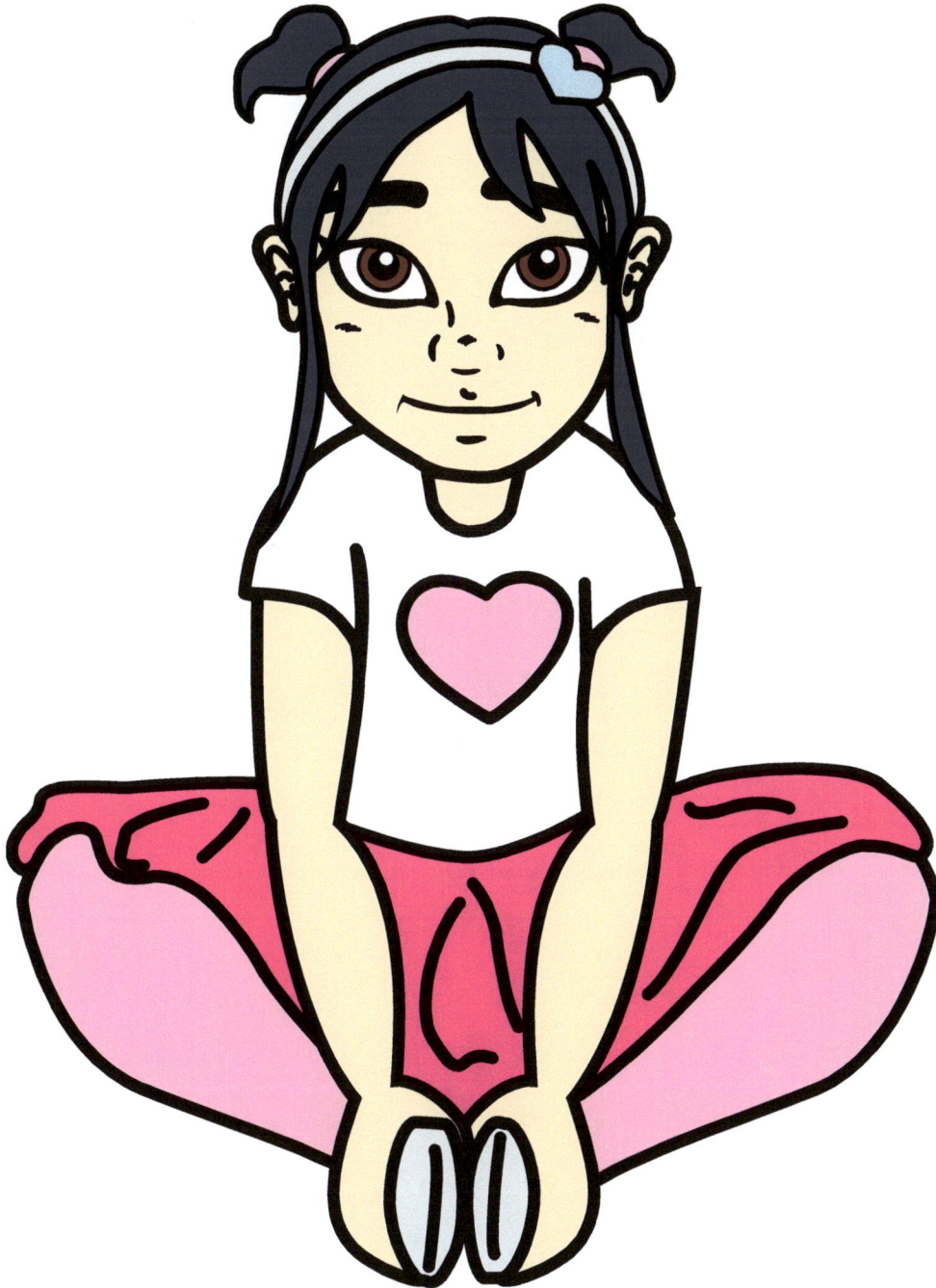

Chair Pose

Stand up straight

Put your feet together

Place your palms together

Reach up tall

Slowly lower your body

Slowly breathe in and out

Hold this pose for 5 seconds

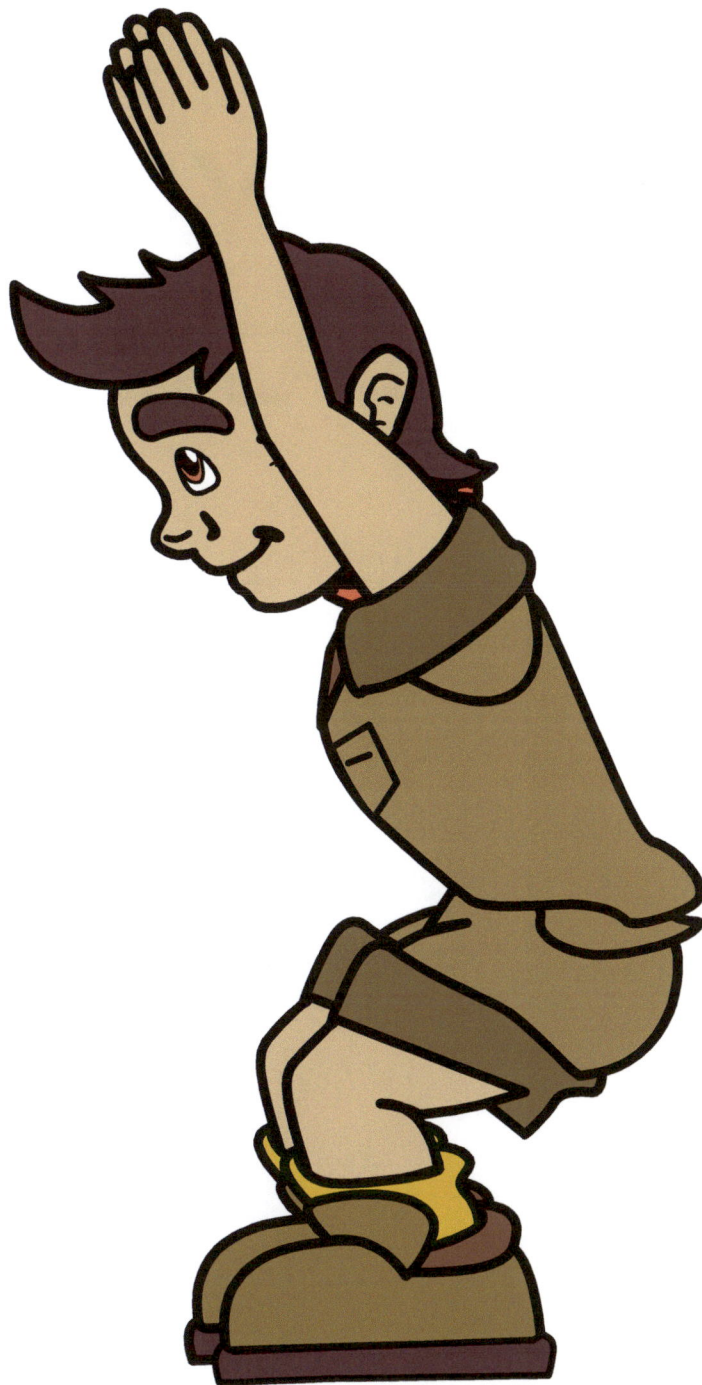

Yoga 25

Downward Facing Dog Pose

Kneel on the floor

Put your palms on the floor

Lift your bottom up

Keep your body strong

Slowly breathe in and out

Hold this pose for 5 seconds

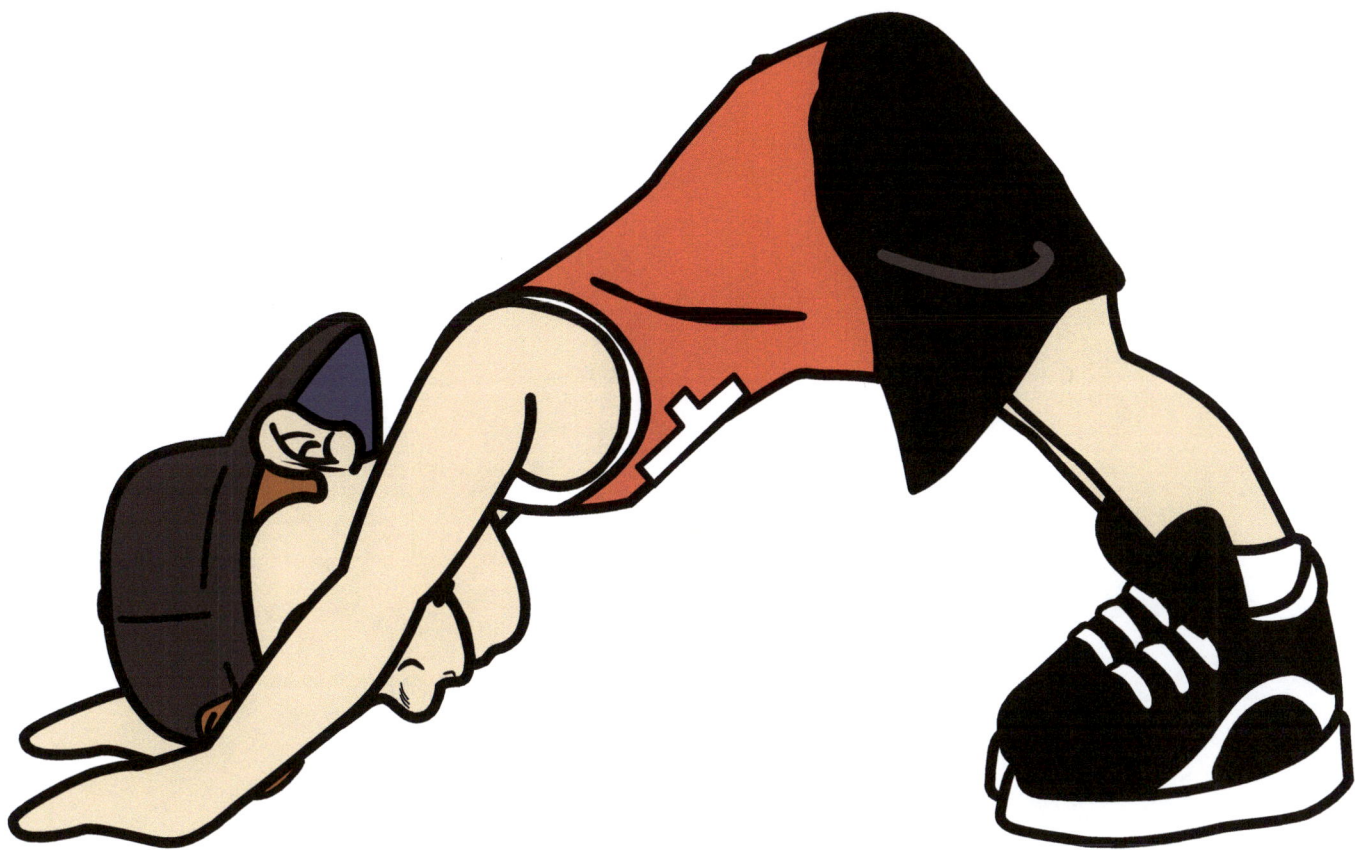

Bridge Pose

Lay on your back

Bend your knees

Slide your feet under your knees

Place your hands beside you

Slowly lift your hips upward

Slowly breathe in and out

Hold this pose for 5 seconds

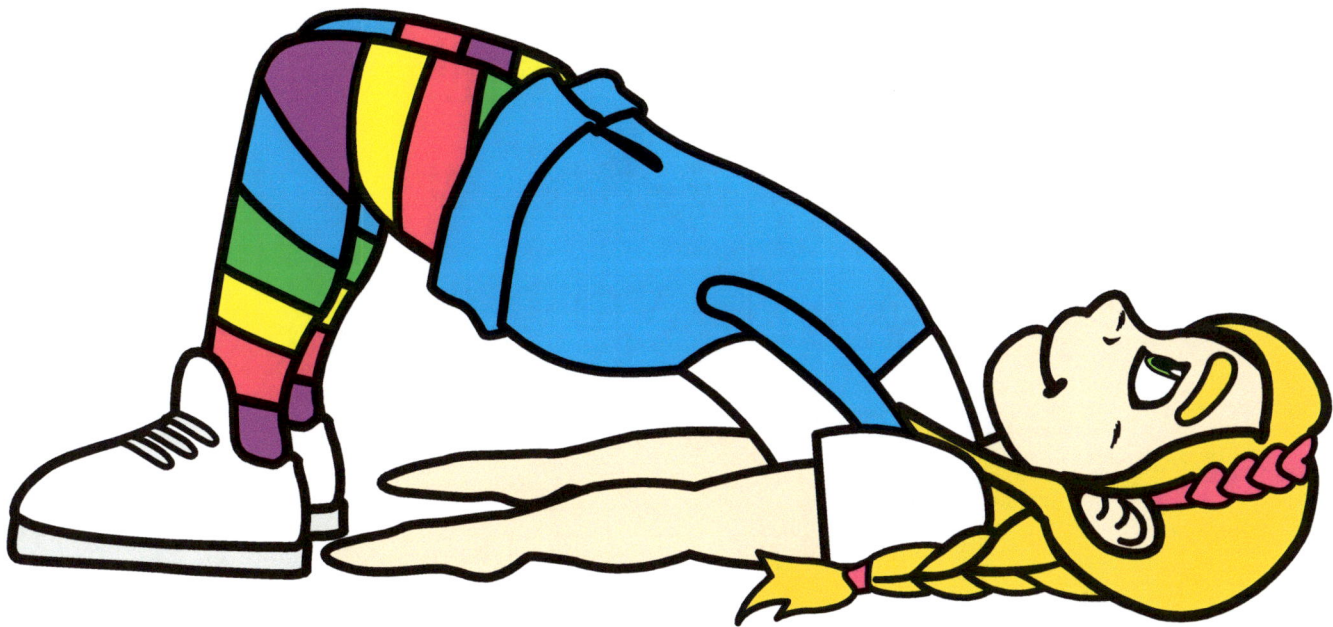

Crescent Moon Pose

Stand up straight
Put your feet together
Reach up high with your palms
Put your palms together
Slowly bend to the left
Slowly breathe in and out
Hold this pose for 5 seconds
Let's do this to the other side

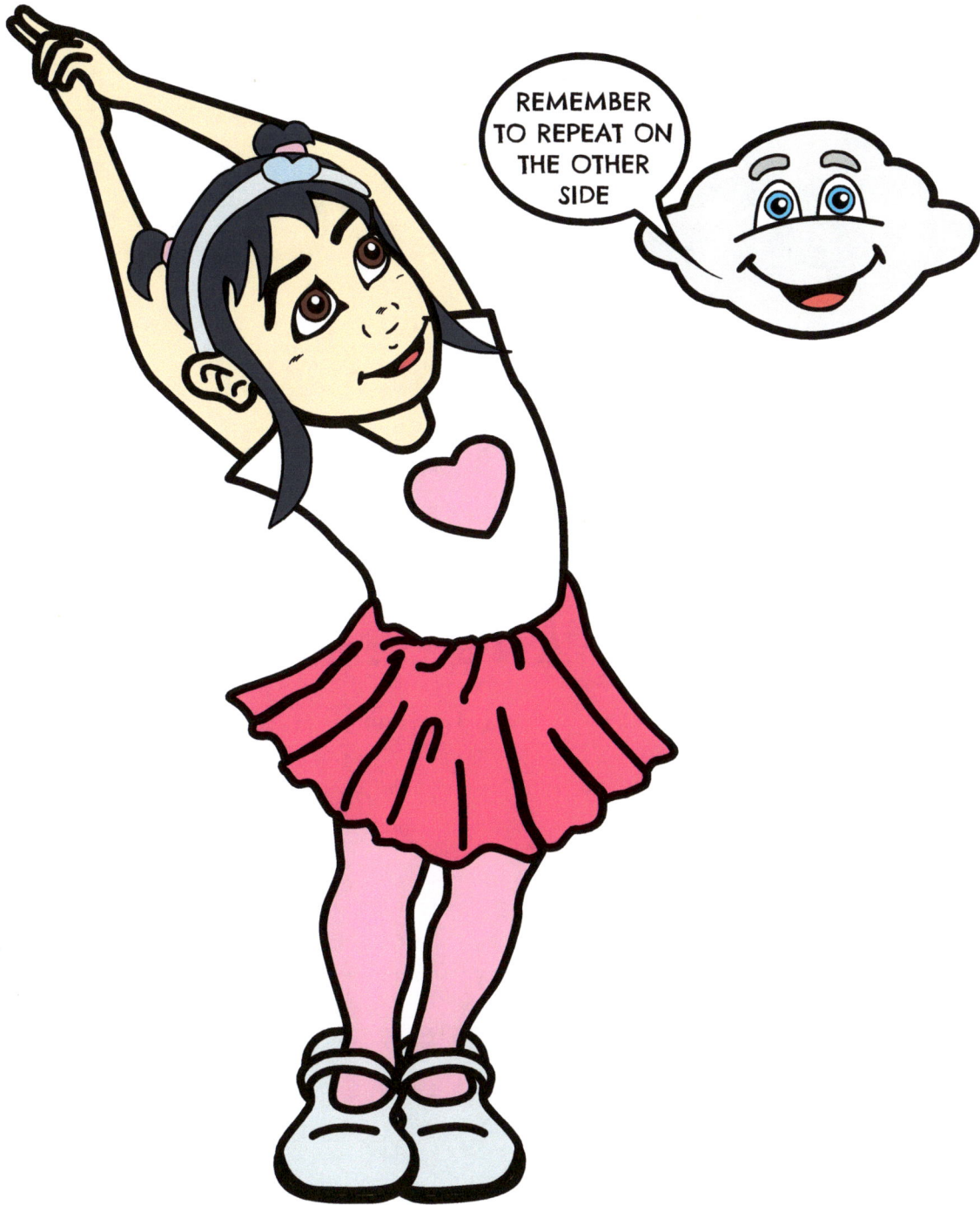

Extended Side Angle Pose

Stand up straight
Twist your body to the left
Take a step to the left
Point your toe
Lower your body
Place your elbow on your knee
Reach your other arm up high to the side
Slowly breathe in and out
Hold this pose for 5 seconds
Let's do this to the other side

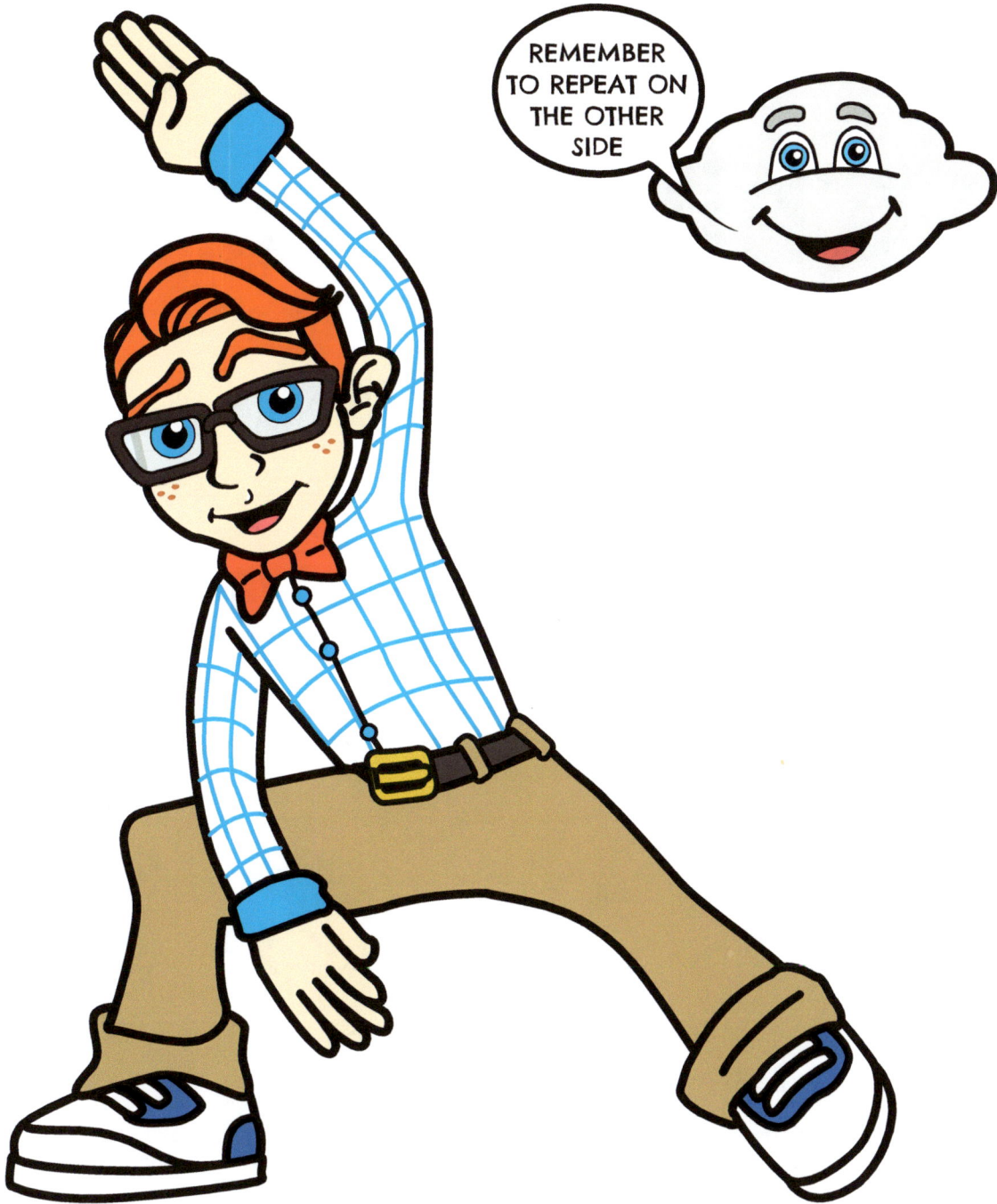

Child's Pose

Kneel on the floor

Stretch your arms up

Slowly lower yourself to the floor

Hold it right there

Slowly breathe in and out

Hold this pose for 5 seconds

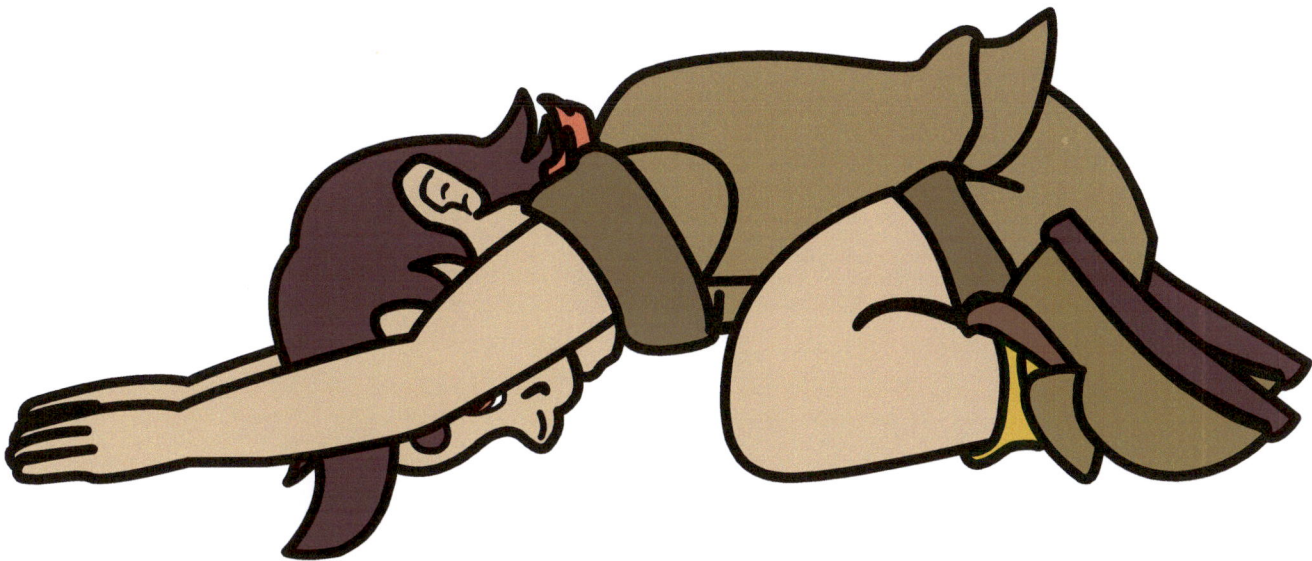

Keep an eye out for the rest of the series

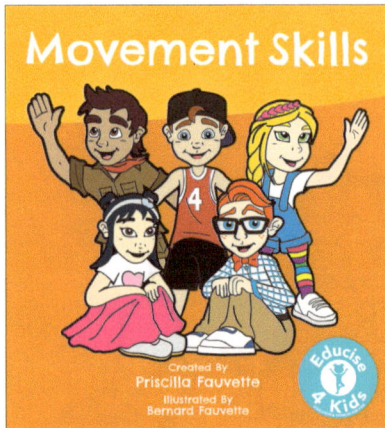

Movement Skills

Created By
Priscilla Fauvette
Illustrated By
Bernard Fauvette

Educise 4 Kids

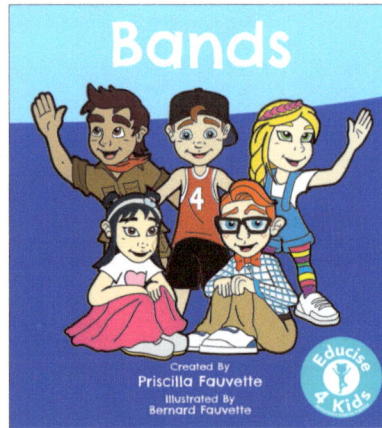

Bands

Created By
Priscilla Fauvette
Illustrated By
Bernard Fauvette

Educise 4 Kids

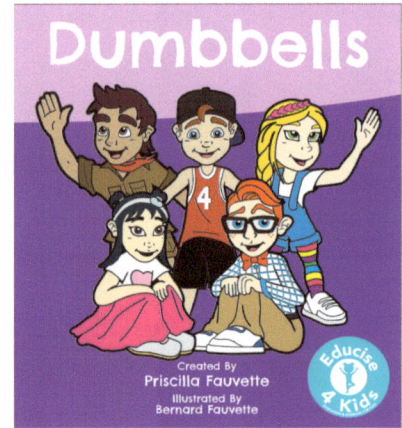

Dumbbells

Created By
Priscilla Fauvette
Illustrated By
Bernard Fauvette

Educise 4 Kids

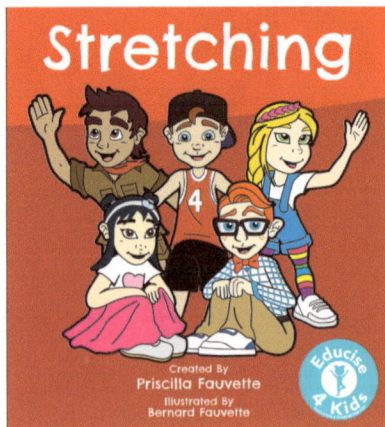

Stretching

Created By
Priscilla Fauvette
Illustrated By
Bernard Fauvette

Educise 4 Kids

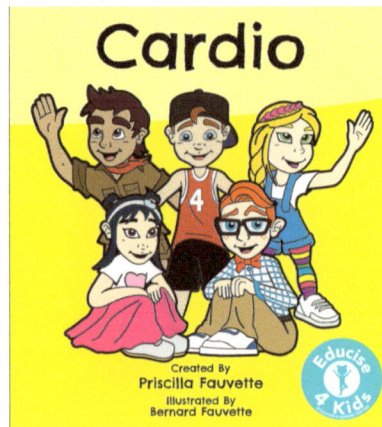

Cardio

Created By
Priscilla Fauvette
Illustrated By
Bernard Fauvette

Educise 4 Kids

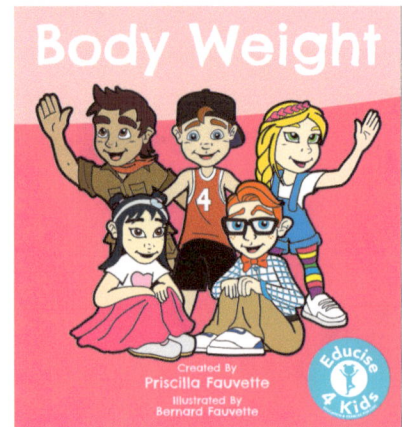

Body Weight

Created By
Priscilla Fauvette
Illustrated By
Bernard Fauvette

Educise 4 Kids

www.ingramcontent.com/pod-product-compliance
Lightning Source LLC
Chambersburg PA
CBHW061137030426
42334CB00003B/80